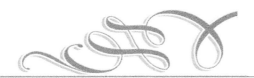

All About Grandma Memory Journal

(I didn't know that about you!)
Prompted Journal for Grandma

Megan Adams

In Loving Memory of my Grandmother. There is no greater gift than to be loved, but to be loved by a grandmother is a precious comfort. Grandma, although I was one of many grandchildren, you always made me feel special. I will always remember you for quietly showing your faith in God through your actions and for pretending you weren't the one who farted in the car.

Journals available by Megan Adams
I didn't know that about you!
Series of Prompted Journals

All About Mom Memory Journal
Prompted Journal for Mom

All About Dad Memory Journal
Prompted Journal for Dad

All About Grandma Memory Journal
Prompted Journal for Grandma

All About Grandpa Memory Journal
Prompted Journal for Grandpa

All About Grandma Memory Journal
(I didn't know that about you!)
Prompted Journal for Grandma

Copyright © 2017 by Megan Adams.
All rights reserved. This book or any portion thereof
may not be reproduced or used in any manner whatsoever without
the express written permission of the author.

First Printing, 2017
ISBN 978-1542990820

_____

_____

_____

Use this journal to capture the memories that make you so special to your family. The journal is divided into sections with empty pages at the end of each if you wish to tell extra stories or include other information. Fill out as much or as little as you want. Change the questions to fit your life and add topics that are specific to you. I hope that this journal brings back special times and thoughts for you. Your family will always treasure your memories. Enjoy.

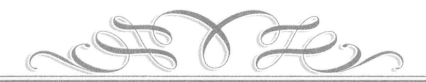

Table of Contents

Childhood Memories
- Family life — 2
- Food and Meals — 10
- School — 12
- Under the weather — 16
- Grandparents — 18
- Holidays — 20
- Fun — 24

Adult Memories
- Work — 32
- Travel — 34
- Adventure — 36
- Love — 38

Parenting
- Babies — 46
- Children — 48

The World Around You
- Fashion — 58
- Food — 60
- Events — 62
- Technology — 64

About You
- Beliefs — 74
- Thoughts — 76
- Advice — 82

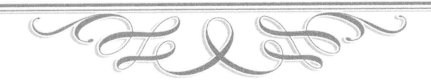

Childhood Memories

Childhood Memories

Who did you live with as a child? (list relatives full names...for siblings note how much older and/or younger each was):

_____
_____
_____
_____
_____
_____
_____
_____
_____
_____
_____
_____
_____
_____
_____
_____

When and where were you born?

_____
_____
_____
_____
_____

Family Life

What did your Mom and Dad do for a living?

_____
_____
_____
_____
_____
_____
_____
_____
_____
_____

What was your bedroom like? Did you share it? Decorate it?

_____
_____
_____
_____
_____
_____
_____
_____
_____

Childhood Memories

What kind of chores did you have?

_____
_____
_____
_____
_____

Did you get along with your brothers/sisters? Was there a favorite?

_____
_____
_____
_____
_____

What kind of vehicle did your family own? Where did you sit?

_____
_____
_____
_____
_____

Family Life

Did you consider your family poor, average, rich?

_____
_____
_____
_____
_____

Were your parents strict? What did you get for a punishment?

_____
_____
_____
_____
_____

Did you have any pets?

_____
_____
_____
_____

Childhood Memories

What was the best and worst trait about your Mother?
_____
_____
_____
_____
_____
_____
_____
_____
_____
_____

What was the best and worst trait about your Father?
_____
_____
_____
_____
_____
_____
_____
_____
_____
_____

Family Life

What was the best thing about having siblings? (if you didn't have any, what was best about being an only child?)

_____
_____
_____
_____
_____
_____
_____
_____
_____
_____

What was the worst thing about having siblings? (if you didn't have any, what was worst about being an only child?)

_____
_____
_____
_____
_____
_____
_____
_____
_____

Childhood Memories

Where did you live as a child? If you moved what was it like to move to a new place?

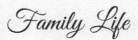

What kind of vacations did your family go on?

What was your best family vacation?

Childhood Memories

List 3 of your favorite home cooked meals...

_____
_____
_____
_____
_____
_____

What was your favorite dessert?

_____
_____
_____
_____
_____
_____

What meal or food was a special treat?

_____
_____
_____
_____
_____
_____

Food and Meals

How often did you go out to eat? Did your family have a favorite?

_____
_____
_____
_____
_____

Did you do any cooking or baking?

_____
_____
_____
_____
_____

What food or meal did you hate as a kid?

_____
_____
_____
_____

Childhood Memories

Did you like school? Was it hard or easy for you?

_____
_____
_____
_____
_____
_____

What kind of school did you attend?

_____
_____
_____
_____
_____
_____

Did you walk or ride a bus? How far was it?

_____
_____
_____
_____
_____
_____

School

What was your favorite subject? Why?

What was your worst subject? Why?

Childhood Memories

What was a typical school lunch like?
_____
_____
_____
_____
_____
_____

Were you in any clubs?
_____
_____
_____
_____
_____
_____

Did you play sports in school?
_____
_____
_____
_____
_____
_____

School

Did you ever get in trouble at school?

_____
_____
_____
_____
_____
_____

How big was your high school?

_____
_____
_____
_____
_____
_____

What did you want to be when you grew up?

_____
_____
_____
_____
_____

Childhood Memories

Did you get sick a lot when you were a kid?
_____
_____
_____
_____
_____
_____

Did you get the measles or mumps?
_____
_____
_____
_____
_____
_____

Did you break any bones?
_____
_____
_____
_____
_____
_____

Under the Weather

Do you have any scars?

Did someone in your family get sick or injured?

What was going to the dentist like?

Childhood Memories

Describe your Grandmother(s):

_____
_____
_____
_____
_____
_____

Did (does) she have a special trait, recipe or tradition?

_____
_____
_____
_____
_____
_____

Please share a special memory of her:

_____
_____
_____
_____
_____

Grandparents

Describe your Grandfather(s):

_____
_____
_____
_____
_____
_____

Did (does) he have a special trait, recipe or tradition?

_____
_____
_____
_____
_____
_____

Please share a special memory of him:

_____
_____
_____
_____
_____

Childhood Memories

Did you celebrate Halloween? How?
_____
_____
_____
_____
_____
_____

Did the toothfairy visit you? Give you money?
_____
_____
_____
_____
_____
_____

Did you get an Easter Basket?
_____
_____
_____
_____
_____
_____

Holidays

What religion were you raised?

_____
_____
_____
_____
_____

Did you/How did you celebrate Christmas?

_____
_____
_____
_____
_____

Did you pray?

_____
_____
_____
_____
_____

Childhood Memories

What was your favorite holiday? Why?

_____
_____
_____
_____
_____
_____

What was a family holiday tradition?

_____
_____
_____
_____
_____
_____

Who did you celebrate important holidays with?

_____
_____
_____
_____
_____
_____

Holidays

How did your family celebrate your birthday? Do you remember any birthday as being extra special?

_____
_____
_____
_____
_____
_____

What was your best birthday present?

_____
_____
_____
_____
_____
_____

What was your favorite birthday cake?

_____
_____
_____
_____
_____

Childhood Memories

Who was your best friend(s)?
_____
_____
_____
_____
_____

What did you and your friends do for fun?
_____
_____
_____
_____
_____

Did you have sleepovers? A secret hideout?
_____
_____
_____
_____
_____

Fun

What was your favorite toy?

_____
_____
_____
_____
_____

What indoor games did you play?

_____
_____
_____
_____
_____

What outdoor games did you play?

_____
_____
_____
_____
_____

Childhood Memories

Childhood Memories

Childhood Memories

Childhood Memories

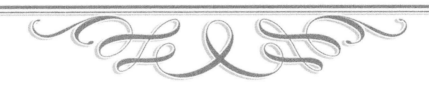

Adult Memories

Adult Memories

What was your first full time job?
_____
_____
_____
_____
_____
_____

If you could have had a different career what would it be?
_____
_____
_____
_____
_____
_____

What types of Education/Training have you had?
_____
_____
_____
_____
_____
_____

Work

What was something you're proud of regarding work?

_____
_____
_____
_____
_____
_____

What was your best job?

_____
_____
_____
_____
_____
_____

What was your worst job?

_____
_____
_____
_____
_____

Adult Memories

What are the two best places you have visited?
_____
_____
_____
_____
_____
_____

Where do you wish you had gone, or would like to go?
_____
_____
_____
_____
_____
_____

Do you wish you had traveled more? If yes, where?
_____
_____
_____
_____

Travel

What was the worst place you visited?

_____
_____
_____
_____
_____
_____

If you could have a second home anywhere, where would it be?

_____
_____
_____
_____
_____
_____

Do you prefer exciting or relaxing vacations?

_____
_____
_____
_____
_____
_____

Adult Memories

What are the two most daring, adventurous or dangerous things you've done?

Adventure

What interesting activities have you tried?

_____
_____
_____
_____
_____
_____
_____
_____
_____
_____

What are two unusual foods you've tried? Were they better or worse than you expected?

_____
_____
_____
_____
_____
_____
_____
_____
_____
_____

Adult Memories

Who was your first crush/love?

_____
_____
_____
_____
_____
_____

How long were you and Grandpa together before you had children?

_____
_____
_____
_____
_____
_____

What is the nicest or most romantic thing Grandpa ever did for you?

_____
_____
_____
_____
_____

Love

What kind of wedding did you have?

_____
_____
_____
_____
_____
_____

Where did you go for your honeymoon?

_____
_____
_____
_____
_____
_____

What was/is the best part about marriage?

_____
_____
_____
_____
_____
_____

Adult Memories

Adult Memories

Adult Memories

Adult Memories

Parenting Memories

Parenting Memories

Did you plan on how many kids you wanted?

_____
_____
_____
_____
_____
_____

What was pregnancy like?

_____
_____
_____
_____
_____
_____

What was childbirth like?

_____
_____
_____
_____
_____
_____

Babies

What did you feed your baby?

___

Who helped take care of your kid(s)?

___

Did you read to your child(ren)?

___

Parenting Memories

Describe three scary events/injuries with your child(ren):

Children

What do you wish you had done more of with your children?

_____
_____
_____
_____
_____
_____
_____
_____
_____
_____

What do you wish you had done less of with your children?

_____
_____
_____
_____
_____
_____
_____
_____
_____
_____

Parenting Memories

Do you think you were strict, moderate or easy on your kid(s)?

_____
_____
_____
_____
_____
_____

Do you think you expected too much/just right/not enough of your child(ren)?

_____
_____
_____
_____
_____
_____

Were you overprotective?

_____
_____
_____
_____
_____

Children

What did you enjoy doing with your kids?
_____
_____
_____
_____
_____
_____

What games did you play with your child(ren)?
_____
_____
_____
_____
_____
_____

What was the hardest thing about raising kids?
_____
_____
_____
_____
_____

Parenting Memories

Parenting Memories

Parenting Memories

Parenting Memories

The World Around You

The World Around You

Share a memory about the following fashions:

Bell bottoms or designer jeans

_____
_____
_____
_____
_____
_____

Leg warmers or shoulder pads

_____
_____
_____
_____
_____
_____

Hot Pants, mini skirts or tie-dye

_____
_____
_____
_____
_____
_____

Fashion

Platform shoes, trendy boots or clogs

_____
_____
_____
_____
_____
_____

Favorite fashion trend?

_____
_____
_____
_____
_____
_____

Least favorite fashion trend?

_____
_____
_____
_____

The World Around You

Share a memory of the following....

Fondue, Velveeta or Cheez Wiz

_____
_____
_____
_____
_____

Oleo, lard, margarine or butter

_____
_____
_____
_____
_____

TV dinners or breakfast cereals

_____
_____
_____
_____
_____

Food

Candy cigarettes or penny candy

_____
_____
_____
_____
_____
_____

Glass Coke bottles or soda fountains

_____
_____
_____
_____
_____
_____

Cream puffs, baked Alaska or ice cream trucks

_____
_____
_____
_____
_____
_____

The World Around You

How were you or your family affected by, or what memories do you have of...

Gas Shortage

_____
_____
_____
_____
_____
_____

Wars/World Conflicts

_____
_____
_____
_____
_____
_____

Natural Disasters

_____
_____
_____
_____
_____
_____

Events

9/11

_____
_____
_____
_____
_____
_____

Cold War/Nuclear Fears

_____
_____
_____
_____
_____
_____

_____ (one that stands out in your memory)

_____
_____
_____
_____

The World Around You

When did you get your first cell phone? What kind was it?

_____
_____
_____
_____
_____
_____

Describe your first car:

_____
_____
_____
_____
_____
_____

How did you listen to music growing up?

_____
_____
_____
_____
_____
_____

Technology

How did you watch movies growing up?
_____
_____
_____
_____
_____

When did you get your first computer?
_____
_____
_____
_____
_____

How did you look up information in High School?
_____
_____
_____
_____
_____

The World Around You

What was your experience or memories for the following?

VHS, Betamax Tapes

_____
_____
_____
_____
_____
_____

TV Antennas, remote controls

_____
_____
_____
_____
_____
_____

Computer floppy disks (8 inch, 5.5 inch, 3.5 inch)

_____
_____
_____
_____
_____
_____

Technology

Music cassette tapes, albums

_____
_____
_____
_____
_____
_____

Pagers, fax machines

_____
_____
_____
_____
_____
_____

Rotary phone, answering machine

_____
_____
_____
_____
_____

The World Around You

The World Around You

The World Around You

The World Around You

About You

About You

Do you believe in the following? Have you ever experienced anything related to these?

Miracles

Karma

Ghosts

Beliefs

Aliens

_____
_____
_____
_____
_____
_____

Guardian Angels

_____
_____
_____
_____
_____
_____

Love at First Sight

_____
_____
_____
_____
_____

About You

List 2 skills or talents that you are glad you have:

_____
_____
_____
_____
_____

If you could be any age again, what would it be?

_____
_____
_____
_____
_____

What three characteristics would you like people to think of you as?

_____
_____
_____
_____
_____

Thoughts

Have you had your picture in the newspaper?

___

Have you ever won anything or been awarded something?

___

Have you met any famous people?

___

About You

What days or events in your life have had the most impact on you?

Thoughts

What are three of the nicest things someone has done for you?

About You

What has been your biggest challenge?
_____
_____
_____
_____
_____
_____

What have you disliked about growing older?
_____
_____
_____
_____
_____
_____

What have you liked about growing older?
_____
_____
_____
_____
_____
_____

Thoughts

What do you wish you had known when you were younger?

___

How were things harder growing up then they are today?

___

How were things easier growing up then they are today?

___

About You

What advice do you have about the following:

Friends
_____
_____
_____
_____
_____
_____

Family
_____
_____
_____
_____
_____
_____

Marriage/Love
_____
_____
_____
_____
_____
_____

Advice

Raising Children

_____
_____
_____
_____
_____
_____

Career

_____
_____
_____
_____
_____
_____

Growing older

_____
_____
_____
_____
_____

About You

About You

About You

About You

Made in the USA
Monee, IL
10 December 2022